ITALIA GLAM

BRING ITALIAN GLAMOUR INTO YOUR LIFE

KRISTI BELLE

INTRODUCTION

Ciao bella!

Before you dip into this book (hopefully with an espresso or glass of wine and maybe an anise biscotti), I must make a disclaimer.

I'm not 100% Italian.

Shocking, I know.

I'm only part Italian.

I'm Italian-American.

And I do not live in Italy.

I'm from California but I currently live in Minneapolis.

But I have sought to incorporate Italian values, ideas, and philosophies into my world for my entire adult life.

In addition, I must admit that I have not spent as much time in Italy as I would've liked to at this point in my life.

I still have so much of Italy to explore (see the author's note at the back of this book!)

As I write this, I have only spent time in Rome and Florence.

My excuse is that I'm a city girl so those were the places I wanted to explore first.

Even though my family is from Southern Italy, I have not yet been

INTRODUCTION

there. And in fact, my upcoming trip to Italy is going to be up north (Verona and Venice).

With all that said, I want to make it clear that this entire little gem of a guide is completely my own interpretation of Italian glamor and how to bring that into my world.

I am sharing it with you because I tend to write the books I want to read.

It serves as a guide to how I live my life. A small, rich blueprint, if you will.

The words that follow come from deep in my heart and soul and imagination of how I interpret a glamorous Italian woman lives!

It's compiled from my imagination, but also from movies, books and Italian women I know personally and those I've watched from afar.

It is also a glimpse into my own world and how I seek to embody this attitude in my own life as a single woman of a certain age living in a major metropolitan city.

I'm newly single after being married for 27 years so I have been doing a lot of reinventing myself over the past few months.

Part of that exploration has been getting back in touch with my Italian roots.

When I was growing up my father instilled in me great pride (bordering on arrogance) in having Italian genes. Over my life, I've gone back and forth in how much I pay attention to this Italian side.

For me, it has often meant embracing my effusive, passionate nature. My Italian side is all about this enthusiasm for life.

So the words that follow are really about my own take on being a part Italian woman and how I tap into that side of me to make my life more rich and full.

I hope you turn the pages of this book in that spirit.

And if I've done my job, you will close the cover of this book inspired to create a little Italia Glam in your own life.

Grazie mille for reading!

Kristi Belle

YOUR INNER ITALIAN GIRL

Meet Sofia Rocelli. She is the composite of the Italian women I know. She also is a tiny bit of me.

Let's take a look at a morning in her life.

If you will, indulge me as we both imagine what her Italian life is like and then break it down as to why it exudes glamor and lux. Are you ready? Let's go.

Rome, Italy

Morning

Brilliant morning sunlight spills through the sheer white curtains that separate Sofia's bedroom from her small wrought iron balcony overlooking the heart of Rome.

Sofia can feel the warmth of the sun as it casts a golden beam across her face.

Before she even opens her eyes, Sofia stretches languidly like a cat, pushing her arms and hands above her head and smiling.

Sofia slowly opens her eyes and sees the clock on the wall. Right on time.

She is so in tune with her internal body clock she does not need to set an alarm.

When she is done doing a gentle stretch, she unfolds herself out of her bed and throws a silk pale pink robe over her silk and lace matching nightgown. She slides her perfectly manicured toes into luxuriously soft faux fur slippers and then turns to make her bed.

She, of course, sleeps European style, which means a duvet thrown onto a fitted sheet hugging the mattress. No top sheet. The fitted sheet and the duvet cover are 1,000-thread count cotton and a brilliant white. Because the duvet cover serves as a top sheet, she is able to wash it weekly with the bottom sheet and it has become velvet soft.

She shakes out the duvet and spreads it out on the bed and then does the same with two faux fur throws that go on top of the duvet. One is a pearl gray and the other petal pink. After fluffing her four pillows in their silk pillowcases—silk keeps her hair and skin gorgeous at night—she is done.

Padding into the bathroom, she brushes her hair and teeth.

Then she pulls her hair back and grabs a small cobalt blue vial out of her medicine cabinet.

She uses the dropper to pull out about six drops of the high-quality olive oil into her palms. She rubs them together and then gently pats the oil all over her face, neck, and décolletage.

Then she takes out her marble gua sha and does a quick routine, massaging her lymph nodes, using the curves of the tool to carve out her jaw and cheekbones. Using it to pull the small lines away from her face and nose. A gentle sweep under her eyes and song her neck and forehead.

When she is done, she applies caffeine-infused eye patches under her eyes. (Sofia, if you might have guessed is "of a certain age.")

She will leave the patches on during her exercise and morning routine.

The first thing she does is drink a mug full of a fresh-squeezed lemon with some sea salt ground into it. She drinks with a straw so the acid of the lemon won't erode the enamel on her teeth.

After hydrating, she unrolls a dark gray yoga mat in her living room.

Throughout all of this, she still hasn't turned on any bright lights.

Her living room doesn't get the morning sunlight that her bedroom does, but she has soft pink LED lights that make it bright enough to see.

The kitchen is cheery 24/7 with white fairy lights strung around the cabinets.

Her house remains dim with just these two forms of lights from about 8 p.m. on to help her body prepare for her bedtime.

Her living room is cozy, luxurious and comfortable. Everything in it is pleasing to the touch. She has leather, velvets, faux furs. It is not a large condo and the kitchen and living room are one great room.

The great room is filled with plants and candles and books and mirrors and art.

Turning on some energetic happy music she heads to the yoga mat.

A quick workout of floor exercises to music wakes her up and energizes her. She does sit ups, pushups and some kettlebell exercises to keep her derriere taut. Nothing too strenuous. Just a little daily routine that keeps her in top form.

If the weather is atrocious, she may hit the gym in the building for a 20-minute intensive treadmill walk, but normally she is able to get all her walking in during her day.

Before she sips that first anticipated cup of coffee, she curls herself up in the lotus position and meditates for 10 minutes.

Once she is done, she heads to the kitchen and makes herself a pot of coffee in her stainless steel French Press.

Armed with her mug and pot of coffee, she heads to a comfy chair in her living room and picks up her latest nonfiction book. It is always something she is excited and inspired by. She has an ongoing list of books to read during her morning routine and is never at a loss for what it might be.

She has read books on health, on meditation, on boundaries, on decorating, on relationships, minimalism, philosophy, psychology, child raising (when her kids were at home), wealth, manifestation, style and fashion... the list goes on.

Her only requirement is that it must capture her attention and interest and inspire her to live a better, richer life.

Every morning of her life she reads for at least 10 minutes as she sips her coffee. If it is winter and the sun is not yet up, she will often light a candle for the ambience but also the delicious smells that it spreads throughout her space.

Once her reading is done, she turns on some music that makes her happy (her playlist is updated as needed) and opens her leather journal. She prefers a black Moleskine journal lately with a fountain pen. She fills one journal for each month of the year.

At first, if something she read inspired her enough, she will capture that in her journal. If not, she almost always starts out the journal page with a list of her top three things to accomplish that day.

If she does nothing else but those three things she's killed it.

After a journaling session, she opens her laptop and does a quick financial checkup. She logs what she spends each day and checks her budget and account balances to stay on track.

She's building wealth and paying attention to her financial portfolio every day is a way she shows love for that area of her life.

Once her morning routine is done, she showers and applies her makeup sitting at a small vanity table in her bedroom. She often will light a candle and either put on music or a podcast to listen to as she gets ready.

Her cosmetics are prettily displayed.

Her philosophy for her makeup, is the same one she uses for everything else in her life:

Buy less but buy the best.

Living this way takes some trial and error, but ultimately it is worth it.

In the case of her cosmetics, she has carefully determined which products suit her face the best. Most are higher-end department store brands, but some, such as an excellent eyebrow pencil, are from the drug store. She is not picky about where the product is from as long as it does a wonderful job.

Once her makeup is on, she runs a brush through her hair (she washed it the night before to save time) and gets dressed for the day.

Her wardrobe is a wonder to behold.

She splurged on velvet hangers that help her keep her clothes free of pulling, snags, or tears.

Her closet is organized so she can see all her clothes at a glance.

It took several months and many trials and errors but she invested time into creating a uniform of sorts. She chose a "uniform" that suits her lifestyle, budget, and figure, flattering the parts of her body that she loves the most.

For work she has decided on sleek slim black pants that hug her curves. She has them in different weights of wool, in velvet and in leather. They all have the same flattering cut that hugs her derriere—which she has determined is what of her best features and worth showing off—and lengthens her legs by their length, since she believes her legs aren't as long as she'd like them to be.

For going out, she has a variety of sexy and cute tops to wear but for work, she wears a form fitting crew neck top. The top comes in a variety of colors and she has it in both short- and long-sleeved. She has a few different blazers to wear over the tops—a heavy wool, a summer weight wool, a velvet, a silk. They are all in neutral colors, either black, gray, or navy.

She packs a silky camisole and some heels in her work bag and heads back to the kitchen.

There, she packs a glass container that contains her lunch. She meal preps on Sundays so on this Monday, there are five identical containers that she can choose from.

Each one contains vegetables, a protein and often a side item. Sometimes it's broccoli, chicken, and rice. Other times it's a leafy salad with couscous and salmon. She loves bread but usually saves that for the weekends or nights she goes out to dinner with friends. She also has a container at work where she keeps dark chocolate bars and a mini French press. After her lunch, she will make an espresso and nibble on a square of dark chocolate.

Slipping her high-heeled boots on, she grabs her bag and her house keys.

With her bag packed she throws her trench coat over her arm in case it's not as warm as it seems outside and heads out the door.

Her first stop is the local coffee shop, which is only a block down from her apartment.

It is her first interaction that day with other people. She gathers herself first.

Sofia pauses in the doorway before she enters the cafe.

Behind her massive dark sunglasses—Versace of course—she takes in the room at a glance.

Instinctively she taps into her main character aura and pulls all four corners of the room to her in an invisible display of feminine energy at its best.

Only then does she sashay into the room. She walks with her hips in a slow and sultry manner. She does not lead with her torso and upper body. And she does not rush.

If she were not in Rome, say she was in New York City, she would stand out as she walked down the sidewalk. There, like in Rome, you can find some of the most startling stunning women in the world. But in New York many of those women are tapped into their masculine energy and strut down the street like feathered Cornish cocks, daring anyone to mess with them or get in their way.

Do not blame them. This is how they have learned to survive and conquer the world of men. We love them but are sad that they may have lost touch with their feminine side through no fault of their own.

But here, in Rome, the Italian women are so in tune with their feminine energy that they exude both glamor, confidence, and sophistication without losing an ounce of their innate power.

In fact, they are some of the most powerful women on earth.

Their earthy sexiness coincides with their iron hand at ruling their families.

Once she sidles up to the bar, amid admiring glances, she orders a macchiato. It is the one and only time all day she does not drink her espresso black. She also orders a *maritozzo*, a sweet roll filled with cream.

Instead of getting the pastry to go, she sits at a small cafe table on the sidewalk outside and leisurely eats it while she sips her coffee, relishes the sun shining down on her face and watches passerby.

She has made sure to build this relaxing moment into her work schedule. She doesn't want to rush her morning. Or even her day for that matter. So she eats her pastry and sips her macchiato.

The two items will tide her over until her late lunch.

When she is done, she begins her walk to her office.

After greeting a few colleagues, she settles in at her desk and turns on her computer.

SOFIA'S LIFE: MORNING BEHIND THE SCENES

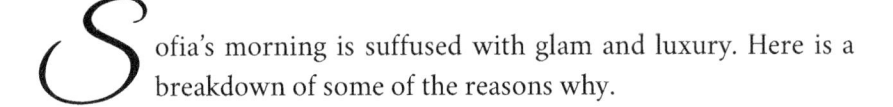

Sofia's morning is suffused with glam and luxury. Here is a breakdown of some of the reasons why.

- She respects and adheres to her natural biological clock when it comes to her bedtime and waking time. She is educated about circadian rhythm and makes sure to keep a consistent sleep schedule so she wakes up energized and joyful instead of tired, crabby, and rushed.
- She prioritizes herself above everything else. For Sofia, this means she makes her sleep schedule so that she is able to wake up and do some daily self-care every single day before she turns her day over to someone else at a job. These 90 minutes in the morning are what sets her entire day up for success. If she has done nothing else that day, she has at least done some self-care in the morning with her rituals and routines and this lays the foundation for greater success throughout her day. If she waited to do these things later in the day, there is a good chance they wouldn't happen. Experience has shown that most people who do this get caught up in their day and these items fall off. By grounding

herself this way every morning she is able to make incremental, but critical gains in her life.
- By buying less but the best, she isn't overwhelmed by choices every morning. For instance, her careful thought into cultivating her wardrobe means she has a standard uniform that she knows fits well, looks good, and makes her feel like a million bucks so she doesn't waste time trying on outfits and figuring out what works. She's already spent time on the back end doing this and now just chooses an outfit from her carefully curated closet.
- She has organized her life such that everything she does in the morning before work takes minimal time. She believes in the Minimum Effective Dose strategy, which means that she has researched what amount of effort yields the maximum result. For instance, studies have shown that the most health benefits from walking are attained at a mere 20 minutes of daily walking. So she does her 20 minutes outside or on the treadmill each day and doesn't worry if it's raining that day and she doesn't walk any more. And her set routines for getting ready are so ingrained that they can be done ahead of time. It's all about having a disciplined life and daily routine. Her home is kept neat and tidy and everything has its place so she is not going to be late to work searching for her trench coat or house keys. She has organized her life and home to be of maximum efficiency so she can spend time and linger over the things in her world that move the needle, such as reading that fascinating book on building wealth every morning and taking notes on how to implement that into her own financial portfolio.
- She infuses even the most mundane daily tasks with meaning by lighting a candle and playing her favorite music. For next to nothing, she can create a glamorous atmosphere in her home.
- Because she is so organized, she has time— and therefore takes the time—to savor the simple pleasures such as that

first sip of coffee and using a fountain pen to write in her Moleskine journal. She splurges on the little things that bring her daily pleasure such as her favorite coffee beans, brand of journal and the fountain pen she bought herself for her 40th birthday.

SOFIA'S LIFE: AFTERNOON

After her leisurely morning start, Sofia's day gets busy quickly (one reason she sets aside time in the morning just for her) and she works straight through until 2 p.m. when she stands, stretches, and goes to retrieve her lunch out of the office break room refrigerator.

She takes it to an outdoor deck where she settles in at a picnic table and slowly enjoys her meal while reading a fiction book she keeps tucked into her work bag.

She briefly checks her phone for anything important—such as a message from her adult children—but then sets it back down.

When she is done eating, she returns to the kitchen and washes her container as water boils on the stove. She makes a press pot of espresso and takes that and her chocolate back to her desk or back to the deck if she has time.

Back at her desk, she works steadily until seven.

It is summer so it is still light outside when she trades her sensible heeled boots for the stiletto sandals she had tucked into her work bag. She takes off her form fitting black top and slips on the lacy camisole before pulling her black blazer back on.

She freshens up her makeup and instead of her flesh colored

lipstick, swipes some bright red color on her lips, fluffs her hair and heads to a nearby restaurant to meet some girlfriends for drinks and dinner. Because her work bag is already filled, she leaves her boots under her desk. She will wear flats to work the next day and then tuck those into her bag and wear her boots to walk home since she doesn't have plans the next night.

SOFIA'S LIFE: AFTERNOON BEHIND THE SCENES

While Sofia's afternoon is a grind—for the most part. She still manages to balance working really hard with carving out time for herself. Here is a breakdown of some of the reasons why.

- She prioritizes taking a lunch break. It doesn't matter how busy she is, she will leave her desk and her office to eat lunch. On a less busy day, she might take her lunch out to a park across the street but because she is on a tight deadline for a project, she sticks to an hour lunch and stays within the building. Even so, she makes sure she eats in a pleasant atmosphere to her—outside.
- On most days, she combines eating alone with something she considers a small luxury, reading an engaging fiction book. Some of her colleagues who sit outside at the picnic table might scroll their phone the entire time, but she would rather do something that she considers a treat, which is reading. A woman who always sits nearby does a little crocheting on a baby blanket after she eats. A man who

often comes out to the deck for his lunch plays online chess. For Sofia, this precious time is well spent reading a book set in ancient Egypt and taking her away to that magical world for a few minutes.

- By making sure she has a healthy lunch consisting of vegetables and protein, Sofia ensures that any afternoon slump she might experience after eating is minimal. And that is helped by the small treat she builds into her every day, a small square of dark chocolate to be savored with espresso. On less busy days, she will come back up to the deck and enjoy those treats outside, but on this day she doesn't mind having them at her desk because she has a project she wants to finish before she leaves the office that day.
- By adjusting her work hours to start later in the morning and work until 7 p.m., she never feels rushed during her work day. She comes in energized and ready to go and is able to sustain that level of energy throughout her afternoon.

SOFIA'S LIFE: EVENING

Dressed for a night out, Sofia adds one last, finishing touch and spritzes herself with some of her signature perfume from a travel-size cylinder she keeps in her bag.

Before she steps outside of her building into the night, she does a mental adjustment.

In her mind, she sheds Sofia the Boss Babe, and slips on Sofia the Hot Babe.

And, indeed, from the minute she steps foot outside her work, heads turn.

She is projecting a confident, sophisticated, feminine and sexy woman out on the town.

The transformation works so well that her office buddy, Rafa, does a double take when he absent-mindedly stops to hold the door for the person behind him—which is Sofia.

She gives him a slight Mona Lisa smile and strides past.

"Don't break any hearts tonight," he says laughing.

"No promises," she flings over her shoulder.

Rafa and Sofia are both divorced and tried dating once but found they were much better as friends. He sometimes joins her for lunch on the terrace but only if he's invited. He knows that if anything, Sofia has firm and gentle boundaries and protecting her "Me Time" is one of them. He is not offended but rather respects that she knows how important this time is to keep her balanced.

In fact, he does much of the same, but his lunch time escape is to the building gym during lunch with his noise-canceling headphones to have his own "Me Time."

As Sofia walks down the sidewalk she doesn't rush. She walks in a way that projects her feminine energy—by moving forward with her hips and legs. The focus on her lower body instead of her torso and shoulders gives her that feminine energy.

Her posture is impeccable. And although her heels are high, they are a pair that she can walk in easily because she knows nothing destroys la bella figura more than a woman walking awkwardly, clumping around in the wrong heels. That is the epitome of *bruta figura* to most Italian women. If you can't walk gracefully in your heels, then stick to flats or find the right high-heeled shoes that work for you.

Sofia knows that for her a slight platform on a heel makes all the difference in walking like a ballerina vs. a construction worker.

As she passes people, Sofia has a slight smile on her face. Her smile will widen if she sees another woman. At this stage in her life her confidence is off the charts and she goes out of her way to be open to other women in all ways.

But if a handsome man is in front of her, she won't hesitate to meet his eyes with a knowing look that shows her appreciation.

Tonight during her walk, one man meets her gaze. He's walking with another man and they are having a seemingly intense conversation.

When his eyes land on Sofia, he pauses for a half second in his conversation but then she is gone and he continues talking.

He is so attractive that she is tempted to do a half turn and watch him walk away. But she won't. She never chases. She only attracts.

As a woman of a certain age, she knows that admiring glances from younger men are often just that—a person admiring another person. But sometimes there is more—a phone number exchanged and a date.

Sofia is not interested in a boyfriend right now unless the man is exceedingly exceptional. But she does enjoy dating a variety of men. It's not exactly a roster, she tells her friends. It's more like a rotating list of men she is seeing. Depending on how the men meet her expectations, they can move up on the list or drop off altogether.

She looks at it like an interview process. Each date is a chance to see if the candidate is a good fit for the position of boyfriend.

Tonight, her friends have invited a single man who they think Sofia might like.

She's hopeful but has zero investment in the outcome.

Finally, she is at the restaurant.

Her friends wave her down. They have secured a table outside.

The area is cordoned off with a small fence which has fairy lights entwined in it.

She heads into the restaurant and strides through to the patio.

After she and her friends greet each other with kisses on the cheek and hugs, she is introduced to Paulo.

He's seated across from her and seems interesting. He's incredibly attractive but so are a lot of men on her roster. He's going to have to demonstrate something special if she kicks someone off her roster to date him.

The dinner and conversation is top notch, though.

Her friends are well educated and witty and she finds herself engaged in passionate, heated conversations about films, books, sex, and politics.

Nothing is off limits.

She carefully listens to Paulo's opinions. So far he has not disqualified himself. His opinions that differ from hers are not deal breakers.

During a lull in conversation she asks him some questions. She is trying to find out if he's worth talking to more at a later date. Skillfully she unearths that he is ambitious and has a good job. First hurdle cleared.

She can save the other fact-finding questions for another time.

Because now the restaurant is kicking them out. It's 1 in the morning.

They've gone through several bottles of wine and polished off a feast.

After a quick espresso and shared desserts, Sofia and her group stand to leave.

A few of her friends are going to an after-hours club. After all, it is a Friday night and nobody has to work the next day.

But Sofia has plans to meet a man for coffee the next day and has weekend chores she would like to finish first. In addition, unless it is a very special occasion, say a concert or opera or festival, she is very strict about keeping to her sleep schedule.

She tells them she'll catch them next time but that she hopes they have fun.

The rest of the group discusses how to get to the club a few miles away.

While this happens, Sofia takes out her phone to call for a ride. It's late and although the neighborhood is safe, she doesn't take chances.

One of her male friends says, "Do you want me to walk you home?"

Sofia is about to explain she's calling for a ride when Paulo is suddenly at her side "I'd love to walk you home."

He is vetted by her friends so she knows he's not dangerous. She pauses a moment and then agrees.

They have a lively conversation during the walk home.

In front of her apartment building she turns to him and thanks him for walking her home safely.

He asks for her number. She gives it to him and leaves.

So far he's passed the test. He didn't ask to come inside. He didn't try to kiss her so soon.

Once she's in her place, she receives a text.

It's Paulo.

He asks if she is free next week to go to dinner.

She tells him she's not but would be available for dinner the following Thursday.

He immediately responds with a text saying he'll reach out to her with details the next day.

Satisfied, she sets her phone down and gets ready for bed.

SOFIA'S LIFE: EVENING BEHIND THE SCENES

Sofia knows that to be her best self she must make time for pleasure in her life but balance it with the habits that keep her energized and healthy.

Here is a breakdown of how she makes her evening fulfilling.

- She prioritizes time with friends. She knows that good conversation and laughter is one of the small luxuries in life that money can't buy. Years ago, she began actively opening herself up to the sort of rewarding and rich friendships that she knew she would want and need as her children left the next.
- Just like she curated her wardrobe, she has cultivated her friends. Like finding flattering clothes, it took some trial and error. After her divorce her first group of women friends were just what she needed but only for a month or two. She quickly realized that going out every night and drinking was fun at first, but quickly grew old. At first, she thought that maybe seeing these women sporadically would work but then she realized that the focus on alcohol was the

only thing these women had in common with one another. And worse, when Sofia didn't want to drink during their outings, she realized that the friendships between these women were toxic. So she decided it would be better to sit home alone than subject herself to a drunk woman's abusive tirade.

- Finding her core group of friends took some time but after about a year of joining groups such as a film group, a fundraising group to save a historic building, and taking up bocce, she made new friends. It ended up that joining a bocce ball team was the key. The friends she met at the restaurant during the tournaments began meeting outside the games and now, five years later, are a solid, core group of friends who meet out at restaurants but also gather for intimate dinner parties at each other's homes.
- Sofia holds firm to her boundaries. While she is as fun and outgoing as the rest of her friends, she knows that without her eight hours of sleep, she's a wreck the next day. To her, while it would be fun to go dancing, she can do that any night. For now, she wants to keep to her sleep schedule so she has energy for her weekend. She has a list of projects she wants to get done around her apartment that weekend, a fun coffee date planned, plus her regular weekend chores that keep her life smooth. On weekends, she cleans and organizes her apartment, shops, meal preps and generally prepares for her next week so everything can run as smoothly as possible.
- Sofia is pleased that she met a new nice guy but not overly excited about it. She views dating as a way to see if a man meets her expectations before she lets him become too much a part of her life. She doesn't have unrealistic expectations, but does have a set of non-negotiables that she requires if she is going to see a man more than once. She knows that just because she likes a guy doesn't mean he deserves to be in her life. So far, Paulo hasn't done anything

wrong so she is looking forward to getting together with him. She threw the ball in his court and now it's up to him to show that he is the kind of guy who can take charge and plan a real date. Just like Francesco, her coffee date in the morning, has shown that he is punctual, has a good job, is financially stable, and has no addictions or mental health issues. There have not been any red flags, so Francesco is on his third date with Sofia. He asked her for dinner Saturday but she has plans to visit her sister's family that night so she suggested coffee. It was a bit of a test. But he passed. He said while he was disappointed, he understood that he had waited too long to ask her out (Calling on Wednesday).

BREAKING IT ALL DOWN

What did you think about Sofia?

If you are like me, there are some parts of her life that make me green with envy and others that I just can't relate to right now but I'm still able to glean some inspiration for how I want to live my life in the snowy Midwest.

Let's break down three components of Sofia's world that we can incorporate into our own lives: her attitude, her routines and rituals, her beauty, and her style.

ATTITUDE

How do you envision Sofia? Do you see her as a blonde or brunette? Short or tall? Overweight or willowy? Cute button nose or regal Roman one? Full lips or thin? Oval face or square? Long hair or short? Fair skinned or olive?

I would bet that you imagined her as alluring and beautiful no matter what her physical characteristics were.

And that is because of her attitude.

Even in this thinly sketched caricature. she exudes sexiness and confidence.

From the minute she woke up, she knew with certainty that she was the prize. She was worthy. She deserved the attention that men gave her no matter what her size or how her features matched those of what society considered beautiful.

Sofia knows the secret.

The secret to being alluring is your attitude and confidence.

She realized at a young age when she attended a summer music festival with her aunt, who was only eight years older than her, but who was a woman of the world who drew male attention wherever she went.

Sofia was 16 when Adele, 24, took her to a festival in Florence.

One night in their hotel, as Adele spoke to several men on the phone before bed, Sofia asked how she learned how to talk to men and how so many men were in love with Adele.

Her cousin smiled and said, "I'm going to teach you something tomorrow that I wish someone had showed me at your age," she said.

The next day, before they headed to the music festival, Adele took Sofia to a square filled with tourists.

"See that group of men?" Adele pointed. "The ones that are here for a business conference?"

Sofia looked. There were about 50 men standing in one area of the square in front of a hotel.

Sofia nodded.

"I'm going to walk through their group. I want you to watch and report back to me what you see."

Then Adele slipped over to the group and walked through it. A few men acted surprised as she wove through the crowd with her head down, but nobody really acknowledged her. She stopped short of going into the hotel doors and circled back around to Sofia.

When she came back, Sofia scowled. "They ignored you!"

Adele beamed. "Exactly!"

"I don't get it," Sofia said.

"Watch me this time."

Adele headed toward the group again.

This time she paused before she entered their midst. She threw back her shoulders and held her head high and slowly began to walk through the crowd.

Sofia watched in amazement as men stopped mid-sentence to gawk at her aunt. A few men smiled. A few spoke to Adele who gave them a mysterious smile and kept walking.

Suffice it to say when Adele walked in the front door of the hotel, about half of the men in the group were watching her.

When her aunt didn't reappear right away, Sofia circled around the group of men and ran inside the hotel lobby. Adele was sitting in a velvet chair in front of a fireplace talking to a handsome man. When she saw Sofia she winked and patted the seat beside her.

Sofia came and sat. A few minutes later, after asking Adele for her phone number, the man left.

"What did you do differently?" Sofia asked when the man left. "Did you talk to them this time or something?"

Adele smiled and shook her head.

"I know. You stood up straighter," Sofia said.

"A little."

Sofia frowned. "So what did you do differently that last time?"

Adele laughed. "I thought different thoughts."

Staring at her aunt for a few minutes, Sofia was irritated. "That doesn't make sense," she finally said.

"I get that," Adele said. "That's why you need to try it for yourself one day."

"When?" Sofia said, still full of skepticism.

Adele shrugged. "Whenever you want."

"What different thoughts do I think?" Sofia asked.

"That you are the prize."

"Hmmm," Sofia said, still not convinced.

As it turned out, Sofia decided to try it later that day at the festival.

There was a group of teenage boys about her age standing around near a concession booth. She walked through them like she normally would. And like, normal, was ignored.

Then a few minutes later she squared her shoulders and walked by them as if she were the most beautiful woman there. And to her amazement, a few of the boys stared at her. One even smiled.

Nobody asked for her number, but it didn't matter. It worked.

From that day forward, Sofia began to notice women everywhere. She soon realized that a woman who was beautiful but insecure was half as beautiful as she could be if she were confident.

Conversely, Sofia saw that a woman who men fawned over could be less attractive than a woman they ignored because it all came down to how the woman held herself.

It was something nearly indefinable. It was how a woman stood. It was how a woman walked. It was how a woman entered a room. It was how a woman spoke and how she laughed and how she looked at other people.

To sixteen-year-old Sofia, who was just starting to think about dating, the information her aunt had revealed that day had been life changing.

Along with thinking that she was the prize, Sofia began to explore all the different ways her attitude could affect her external world.

From the time she was a teenager, Sofia studied the power of attitude, confidence, and thoughts.

While she was never the most beautiful woman in the room, Sofia always attracted men. After a few not-so-great relationships, she met and married the man who became the father of her children.

It was only after the children were older that she realized she married him because he checked the boxes of what a husband and father should be like but that they did not share a great love or passion. He agreed. They parted amicably and co-parented with mutual respect. She is friends with his new wife.

But while Sofia has had boyfriends and enjoys dating for the most part, she has not found anybody she wants to share her life with. At least not yet. Her last boyfriend was a great guy and they were talking about moving in together but then he got a job in the United States. They broke up but remain friends.

Sofia knows from the minute she wakes up every day to the second she closes her eyes at night, her thoughts can determine her life.

Although she can't change the external world, she can control how she reacts to it and that means everything.

When she wakes up full of joy and grateful, she automatically sees and appreciates the small things in life:

- The warmth of the sun
- That first sip of coffee
- The sweetness of a bite of almond croissant melting on her tongue

- Seeing an elderly couple walking down the sidewalk in front of her holding hands.
- The smell of fresh flowers as she passed the flower market
- Children laughing in the park
- The smile of a stranger as he passes

Her attitude, that life holds a series of small delights around every corner if we just are aware enough to look for them, makes her world rich and magical and glamorous.

ATTITUDE ALSO ENCOMPASSES HER DETERMINATION, perseverance, and discipline.

When things don't go her way, Sofia knows her attitude is what will make the difference between sinking in defeat and using the failure to become stronger.

For instance, when she and several of her colleagues were laid off from her job a few years ago, the distraught group all headed to a local bar where many of them proceeded to drink too much.

One man was near tears as he bemoaned his future saying that his life was now ruined.

When he asked why Sofia was not beside herself, she said that while she had loved her job, and was admittedly frightened about the future, she also was confident that something else was out there for her. She said that she knew she was in for an uphill battle finding a job in that economy but that she had set aside a tiny bit of money for emergencies and would get up each day and treat the task of looking for and getting a job as if it were a job in itself.

And sure enough, six months later, she had a new job but her colleague was still moping around fretting that his life was ruined.

One day Sofia took him aside after he asked her to meet him for lunch and begged her for her advice and opinion. After making sure he really wanted to hear it, Sofia told him if he was walking into a job interview with that attitude of woe-is-me, he was going to strike out. He needed to walk in with confidence that he had what it took to contribute to that company. Instead of thanking her, he got mad and walked out. That was the last time Sofia heard from him.

She believed in offering advice if it were asked for, but that was the extent of it.

It was part of the boundaries she had established to live a serene life. Part of it was that she couldn't control what other people did.

The only thing she could control is her reactions to external events.

It boiled down to attitude.

BEAUTY

Sofia was not traditionally beautiful. But she made the most out of what she was given.

It didn't take an exorbitant amount of money but it did take, like everything else, some trial and error, to figure out what worked.

Once she figured out what her best features were: her lips, her hair and her curvy body, Sofia made sure to emphasize those and downplay the parts she wasn't crazy about. However, there was one exception to this.

From the time she was little, she had a very large Roman nose.

Older women used to tell her mother how Sofia would be pretty if it wasn't for her oversized nose and large lips.

Sofia's mother took her aside later that night.

"That's the same thing they told Sofia Loren and ..."

"Is that why you named me after her?" Sofia asked.

Her mother laughed. "No, I didn't know what you would look like when I named you."

"Oh."

Now, in her 50s, men frequently tell Sofia how much they love her lips and while she doesn't get compliments necessarily on her nose, it is a distinguishing feature that she has grown to love.

She plays up her lips with red lipstick when she goes out on the town, like when she left work to meet her friends for dinner.

Her hair is also one of her favorite features.

Like many Italian-American women, she was born with curly and coarse hair.

But when she became an adult she realized that for Italian women, their hair is an extension of their beauty and exemplifies their style.

Whether it's Isabella Rossellini's sleek and slicked back boy's cut or Monica Bellucci's long luscious locks, hair is part of the Italian woman's sex appeal.

Before Sofia turned 50 she was so busy establishing her career and raising her children that she didn't put as much thought into her hair as she could have. She often pulled it back so it was out of the way and only really styled it if she was going out. She often was so busy that her gray roots would really begin to show before she made it into the salon. And the busier she became the longer the time between haircuts became as well. As a 20-year-old, having clean hair was usually enough.

But one day she looked in the mirror and wondered who that woman was with the bad hair. She looked frumpy. Sofia quickly realized that the older she became the more important it was to make sure her hair looked good. It became a priority.

Her aunt Adele agreed. "The more wrinkles we have on our face, the more important our hair becomes."

The words didn't make that much sense until Sofia began to invest in her hair. Instead of every three months for a cut and color, she went in every six weeks like clockwork.

She also discarded drugstore shampoo and conditioners and invested in higher-end products that combated the natural dryness of hair that came with aging.

Now with regular upkeep, her hair was always smooth, silky and sassy and fit her sophisticated, sexy and powerful look.

Just like she'd dropped the ball on her hair care, she also woke up one day and realized that her makeup regime that had worked on her younger skin no longer worked on aging skin.

Because makeup and skin care is so personal, Sofia went straight to the experts.

She quickly learned that the foundation and powder that had made her skin flawless in her 30s now accented her wrinkles.

She learned a new way to apply makeup and began using new products that made her aging skin supple and glowing.

The secret here was her willingness to adapt and change as her body did.

Creating a beauty regime that might have cost a bit more than she was used to was budgeted for and prioritized because it not only added luxury and glamor into her life, it gave her the self-confidence she deserved.

STYLE

When it comes to their wardrobes, Italian women seem to be born with a desire to find clothing that accent what they've got and Sofia is no different.

And like her Parisian cousins, Italian women like Sofia were raised to buy less than American women. Whether it's hung neatly on a rolling clothing rack, such as in Sofia's Rome apartment or displayed in a walk-in closet in her aunt Adele's villa in Puglia, the Italian woman's wardrobe is curated and refined.

She buys less but she buys the best.

STYLE STAPLES

Sofia's aunt Adele taught her at a young age to save her money and invest in the staple wardrobe items that will last a decade or more.

One of the most important investments, Adele told her, was her shoes.

The first thing many Italians look at on a person is their shoes. Scuffed or dirty or falling apart shoes were *bruta figura* - presenting an ugly figure.

Sofia makes sure to buy less but the best. She invested in stilettos, pumps, kitten-heel sandals, flat jeweled sandals, athletic shoes, walking shoes, ankle boots, knee-high boots and calf-high boots.

All in the finest leather.

Then when it came to the foundation of her wardrobe, she made sure to invest in the following items, buying the best she could afford:

- a few different perfect fitting black pants in various weights for each season
- a few blazers in neutral tones and contrasting weights and materials
- perfect fitting jeans in a few colors and weights.
- High-end blouses in different sleeve lengths and fabrics

SHE ALWAYS BOUGHT these staples in neutral colors but added fun colors in her perfect fitting tops which were cheaper and more disposable and often only lasted a season or two before being replaced.

Because Italian women relish being feminine, Sofia's wardrobe of dresses took up one half of her closet.

UNLIKE THE MORE FRUGAL and modest French girl we always hear about with her one perfect Little Black Dress, Italian women, like Sofia, know that when it comes to a crucial staple like a LBD, it's best to own several so she looks sexy and chic at any occasion.

Many Italian women own at least three black dresses, if not more.

SOFIA HAS CAREFULLY CULTIVATED her wardrobe of Little Black Dresses as follows:

- First, she owns the form fitting Dolce & Gabbana sheath

that fits like a glove but does not reveal an abundance of flesh. A cap sleeve, modest scoop neck and knee-length are appropriate for most occasions. Nobody except her knows it's lined in fabulous leopard print. It makes her feel a little less basic if she's wearing it for a business occasion. At the office, she'll definitely obfuscate the tight fit by throwing on her Elizabeth Beard blazer and simple pumps. If she wants to go straight from the office to a chic bar, she can slip on her stilettos and shed her blazer to reveal a provocative zipper in the back of the dress that unzips from the hem but also from the top of the back.

- For a funeral or a wedding, say, she can whip out her uber classic Diane Von Furstenberg wrap dress. With its ¾ length sleeves and knee-length, it can take her anywhere.

ALONG WITH THOSE two essential LBD's—a black sheath and a flowy wrap-style dress—the Italian woman most likely owns at least one if not all of these dresses. At least Sofia does.

- Bodycon dress. A snug, form fitting, hugging every curve bodycon dress for nights at the club or for a girl's night on the town. If she's younger, this bodycon dress will most likely be sleeveless. If she's a woman of a certain age, it might have long sleeves. No matter what age, there is likely to be a glimpse of cleavage and a bit of leg showing. This dress must hug every curve. And this is where the Italian women, like Sofia, get it right. It doesn't have to cost a fortune for this one. It's not an investment piece. But it might take some time to find the perfect fitting sexy dress.

It doesn't matter a woman's size or shape—there is a form fitting dress out there for everyone. It just might take some time to find it and a teeny bit of help from shapewear, which all of us can Thank God for, right? The secret ingredient an Italian woman has to make this dress work and make herself appealing no matter what societal standards of beauty may call for is confidence. Any woman of any age or size who can pull on a perfect fitting bodycon dress over some shapewear, maybe some tights and some cute heels is going to rock this look!

- Summer Frock A closet essential during the summer is a flowy, feminine summer dress. For those who are younger, it can be a mini dress. For women of a certain age, a midi or knee-length dress is most chic. Again, sleeveless dresses are best for the younger women. This is a general rule of thumb except when it comes to a maxi dress and even then older women who don't live at the gym 24/7 might consider keeping a wrap on or foregoing sleeveless altogether. For this summer dress, a flowy material or linen blend can take you from a stroll along the beach boardwalk, to dinner at a sidewalk cafe or a trip to the farmer's market. The dress works for all worlds and a simple change or shoe and addition or subtraction of accessories will help make it appropriate for all occasions. For instance, a flip flop for the boardwalk stroll—and before you start imagining those cheap plastic beach shoes, we are talking about nice sandals you can slip on with leather soles and leather straps. There are gorgeous ones in leopard print calfskin or adorned with tiny jewels. Remember in Italy your footwear speaks volumes.

- Maxi Dress. Again, black is the chicest way to go here. Another color or even a small pattern on this dress may be cute, but won't have the same effect. What she's going for here is sexy nonchalance. A maxi dress is best when it is sleeveless and flows to your ankles. It can be billowy or it can hug your derriere slightly but it must flow a little when you walk. The chicest way to wear this maxi dress is with minimal makeup and accessories. Either sultry lined kohl eyes and no lipstick or a bright splash of red and no eye makeup. Not both. Jewelry must be kept to a minimum, as well, to maintain the nonchalant vibe. Maybe one chunky bead bracelet and nothing else. Or maybe some long funky earrings and that's it. As for shoes, the go to shoe would be flat leather sandals or leather flip flops.

Sofia didn't go out one day and buy all these dresses at once. She slowly and carefully curated them. She shunned a cheaper wrap dress and saved her Euros until she could easily purchase the Dolce & Gabbana or DVF dress knowing that she would most likely wear them for decades.

PART I

SOFIA LOREN

This Academy-award winning actress epitomizes Italia glam in every possible way.

When the subject comes to sexy Italian women, Sofia Loren owns this title.

After refusing to lose weight or have a nose job, Sofia Loren became famous as an Italian actress and beauty.

Let's look at a few of her secrets:

Loren has always sworn by the following:

- A healthy diet. She eats a well-rounded diet with a focus on the Mediterranean style of eating, which involves lots of fresh fruit and vegetables, beans, whole grains, olives and seafood— and some pasta, of course. Life Magazine quoted Loren as saying, "All you see I owe to spaghetti." However, there is some debate whether this was truly something she said.

- Sleep. Loren prioritizes getting copious amounts of sleep and has said she is in bed by 8pm every night.

- Olive Oil: She once said that in addition to consuming a few tablespoons of olive oil daily, she uses it as moisturizer for her skin and

- Mint leaves. She's said that she has crushed mint leaves to make a paste to apply to get rid of under eye circles.
- Decrease the stress in your life. Loren advises people do whatever it takes including taking a moment to meditate or be grateful to reduce the stress in their lives.
- Attitude. She once said, "Nothing makes a woman more beautiful than the belief that she is beautiful." That's why when her future husband told her to get a nose job for the movie he was casting her in, she flat out refused and said, "'I don't want to touch anything on my face because I like my face. If I have to change my nose, I am going back (home)." People also said her mouth was too big. Again, she didn't listen to them.
- Cold showers. Long before the Wim Hoff method (extolling the benefits of cold showers and cold plunges) Loren began taking 10 minute cold showers to (well basically keep her breasts perky) and give her a boost of energy.
- Walking. Loren has said that women should walk down the street gracefully as if they own it.

MONICA BELLUCCI

This amazing actress is a modern day Sofia Loren.

She was the oldest actress to play a Bond girl and has been named as one of the top 100 hottest women of all time. Her eyes, figure, and hair are admired around the world.

Let's look at a few of her secrets:

Bellucci has said:

- She has trained her hair so she only needs to wash it twice a week so it doesn't dry out and get stripped of its natural oils.
- She tries not to use any heated styling tools or even a blow dryer, which can cause damage, but lets her hair air dry on most days.
- She will apply a dab of olive oil on the tips of her hair to moisturize.
- Unlike Isabella Rossellini, who you will meet below, Bellucci focuses on her eyes more than her lips.
- She knows that drinking enough water is the key to health and good skin and makes sure to get enough each day.
- She makes sure to never go to bed without washing off her makeup.
- Like Sofia Loren, she likes to start out her day with a cold shower.

- She doesn't obsess about her weight and embraces her curves. Like Loren, she says self-confidence is the secret to sexy.

CARLA BRUNI

This singer-songwriter and fashion model was also known for marrying French president Nicolas Sarkozy.

In an article in the Guardian, she said, "I don't go for heels, I never wear make-up. It only seems to enhance age."

Let's look at a few of her secrets:

Bruni has said:

- Because makeup on aging skin can enhance wrinkles, she says as women get older they need a much lighter touch with foundation.
- She believes that a good facial massage rejuvenates her skin.
- She is thoughtful about wearing styles that flatter her body shape. In an article in the Guardian, she said that you can't learn style. You either have it or you don't. She claims not to have it. But said that she knows certain things don't work for her, such as shoulder pads.

ISABELLA ROSSELLINI

*A*nother famous Italian actress and philanthropist who starred in David Lynch's iconic film, Blue Velvet.

She has a very distinctive style she's maintained for decades. Deciding at a young age that her hair was not a strong point (being thin and fine) she chopped it off and has sported a cropped look for most of her adult life.

In addition, Rossellini decided on a uniform decades ago and stocked up on blazers with matching pants. Her suit look is always stylish and appropriate.

Let's look at a few more of her glam secrets:

Rossellini:

- Spends time each day doing a form of self-hypnosis known as positive mirror talk.
- Wears her signature red lipstick to cheer herself up but also to instantly elevate her look for the day.
- Advises women when it comes to makeup to pick one feature and focus on that. (For her, as seen above, it is her lips.)

To be happy, Rossellini says, focus on eating healthy and exercising.

ELIZABETTA CANALIS

Another famous Italian actress and model who also briefly dated George Clooney, in 2010 Maxim named her as one of the 10 most beautiful women in the world.

She has posed nude for PETA and is known for her figure. She had a role on Dancing with the Stars, which ties into her active lifestyle.

Let's look at a few of her habits:

- Prioritizes exercise. Canalis continued to work out during her pregnancies doing Pilates at 7 months.
- She concentrates on eating a healthy diet. Her favorite food is shrimp pasta.
- Has kept her signature style—wearing blazers for decades.
- Makes being active physically but also as an activist speaking out for her causes, attractive.

TEN EASY WAYS TO BRING ITALIAN GLAMOUR INTO YOUR LIFE

1. Buy a pretty colored glass eye dropper vial and add high-quality olive oil to it and then squeeze out a few drops onto your palms. Rub your palms together and then gently pat on face, neck and décolletage.

2. Do a try on session with all your clothes and get rid of any that don't make you feel good and confident.

3. Do the inner work first. Start to project an attitude of confidence from the minute you wake up until you go to bed.

4. Savor the small pleasures in life. Take time to sip your favorite drink instead of gulping it down. Imbue everyday activities with a sense of ritual.

5. Start a gratitude journal where you keep a list of free things that bring joy to your life, such as petting your dog when you wake up, sitting with your face tilted up to the sun during your lunch break, laughing with good friends.

6. Prioritize activities that enhance how good you feel each day, such as getting enough quality sleep, eating nutritious food that gives you energy, and moving your body every day.

7. Buy less but buy the best.

8. Take time to figure out your individual signature style when it

comes to your beauty regimen and your clothing style. Realize it's going to take some trial and error and that it may adapt as you age and your life activities adjust.

9. Focus on eliminating stress and toxicity from your life.

10. Prioritize socializing with other people, especially people who lift you up. Studies show that people who have an active social life live longer.

GRAZIE MILLE

Ciao bella!
Thank you so much for reading my book!

I hope you walked away with, at the very least, a spark of inspiration to bring some Italian glamor into your world.

If we haven't met yet, I'm Kristi. I'm an Italian-American mama and fiction writer who has this super fun secret pen name so I can explore all things feminine. My other books are dark and disturbing and 100% the opposite of what I write under Kristi Belle.

I'm newly divorced and navigating the dating world in my early 50s. I think a book is going to come out of this experience, as well.

I also am a new empty nester. But nowadays what does that mean? I still have two amazing daughters home for the summers, holidays, and many long weekends. Thank God. I love them so much and enjoy their company more than ever!

Because of these two giant life changes (divorce and empty nesting), I have really re-evaluated my life and who I am.

Who am I?

At heart I am an Italian-American woman who wants to live every moment to the fullest.

In my case, this means going to Italy to date men.

Who wants to read a book about that?

Email me at italianscorpioqueen@gmail.com with your thoughts.

In addition, if you like my books, stand by for the next one.

It's called *Simple Pleasures: 101 Ideas to Live a Rich Life*

and you can pre-order it here!

Simple Pleasures: 101 Ideas to Live a Rich Life

BONUS

If you somehow landed here without reading my very first book, La Bella Figura, here is a sneak peek at the beginning of that one, written many many years ago.

La Bella Figura

Italians know how to live. They know how to eke every last drop of pleasure out of life — by enjoying a bowl of pistachio gelato, savoring the feel of an ocean breeze or soaking in the sounds and sights of a night at the opera. They know that the secret to life is in living, not having.

This section is about how to live a life rich in all the things that money can't buy. At the end of your life, what will remain are your memories about how you lived. Make them sweet remembrances. As you live your life, try to ensure you will not have any regrets in how you spend the moments of your life. This is about how you spend your time — because your time is your life.

The first thing you need to do to truly live a life that is in line with *la bella figura* is to make sure you are filling your life "doing" instead of "buying."

For me creating *la bella figura* involves living a life filled with quality over quantity. It is about realizing that "less is more." In its essence, it means valuing experiences over possessions.

This might mean spending your leisure time with friends. For instance, maybe lingering over a cafe au lait at the neighborhood coffee shop instead of meeting that same friend for a shopping excursion at the mall.

It could mean working fewer hours so you have more time to spend with your friends and family or more time to indulge in your hobbies and passions.

Maybe for you, it means living with that old couch so you can spend money on piano lessons for your children. It might mean using the same dishes and silverware you got as a wedding present twenty years ago and splurging on a membership at the opera or instead.

Some friends of mine recently bought a new vehicle that will cost them a bundle in monthly car payments, not to mention insurance. Because I love to travel, I would rather save that monthly payment and spend it on a trip to New York City or — if I save long enough — a vacation to South America. In other words, I would rather drive my trusty, paid-off vehicle — even if it is a beater and the farthest thing from "cool" and spend my money on experiences instead. As long as it gets me from point A to point B, I don't care. I'd rather have more money to spend on an experience I can remember on my deathbed.

It seems many Europeans — especially French and Italians in particular — agree:

"Our next vacation means much more to us than a new car and we would never sacrifice the former for the latter except in case of dire necessity. Give us being and feeling over having any day," — Mireille Guiliano of "French Women Don't Get Fat."

Many Europeans have had to be frugal — credit is not as easily obtained in many countries. And let's face it — you can't spend money you don't have. At least not without credit. It's very Euro chic to only spend what you can afford and to save up for something special. I think when you have to save for something you end up appreciating it more. Having less access to credit encourages Europeans to prioritize their spending for maximum satisfaction.

In "C'est La Vie," author Suzy Gershman writes, "People in France made less money than those in the Unites States but still lived better — partly because of this slower pace of life, partly because of the cultural importance of a good meal (with good wine, bien sur) and partly because with less discretionary income, priorities were better defined. If a French person had to choose between new clothes or a concert ticket, the ticket usually won out."

This "less is more" approach applies to everything you own: kitchen accouterments, knickknacks, bed linens, dishes, art objects and even clothes! I'll go into this more later.

Living *la dolce vita*, which goes hand-in-hand with the *la bella figura* lifestyle, is about taking the time to savor the simple pleasures in life. These small delights are different for everybody. It could be the indescribable joy you get from sleeping in on Sunday morning and then spending the next two hours at your favorite café, sipping your cappuccino and reading the New York Times.

It could be the pleasure you get from preparing a gourmet meal and enjoying it with your family or friends. Maybe for you, it is the satisfaction of working with your hands in the garden, planting flowers and vegetables you will enjoy all summer.

A few of my passions are photography, books, movies and playing chess. I try to devote time to do at least one of these pleasures a few times a week.

I also find one of the simplest and yet most satisfying pleasures in my life is dining *al fresco* at the picnic table on my patio. I set the table with a cheery, bright colored tablecloth and use my good plates and glasses. (Actually, that is another very European concept – using the good stuff and not saving it. I only have the "good" stuff.) Eating outside is a tradition I am establishing for my children. As soon as the warm weather rolls around, they ask me every day if we can eat dinner outside.

Another activity I absolutely love is having friends over for dinner and having good food, wine and great conversation with lots of laughter involved.

Last summer we had my French friend Sophie and her family over. We ate "European" style, starting with small dishes of antipasti, such as olives and pepperoncini to nibble on. The first course was homemade pesto (made from the basil from my garden) on pasta. The second course was pork chops on the grill with roasted asparagus. And, of course we had wine with dinner. After the pork chops, we had a romaine and avocado salad, a cheese course and then Limoncello with the homemade flourless cake my friend had brought.

The dinner stretched for hours and included bouts of conversation and guitar playing out at the picnic table until it was dark and only the candles illuminated our faces. At the end of the night my French friend took me aside and thanked me, saying how much she enjoyed the dinner party and that none of her other American friends had ever done that for her before.

Hosting dinner parties like this is one of my simple pleasures in life. So much so that I've made it part of my self-image. I'll explain.

In the book "Style Statement," by Danielle LaPorte and Carrie McCarthy, one exercise the authors suggest to determine your style is to imagine yourself the subject of a celebrity profile in a magazine. Imagining what picture you want to accompany the article is a great way to help distill your style.

I answered the question by saying that I would want to be photographed either at my kitchen table or at the picnic table in my backyard. I would be wearing a flowered dress. I would be sitting before the remains of a great feast. Friends and family would surround me and my head would be thrown back in laughter. Put food on the table, my family around me, a glass of wine in my hand and that really is me at my happiest.

Take time to really think about what makes you happy -- where and when you are your happiest -- and then make sure you are making time to create those moments in your life.

"The Price of Happiness"

An article from the July 2009 issue of Good Housekeeping magazine sums up a lot of my philosophy and views on money and how to live the *bella figura* lifestyle.

The article basically says that you can find joy, happiness and contentment no matter what your income is.

But you have to think carefully about how you spend your money to make this happen.

"The golden rule: Devote your dollars to things that further your goals and beliefs," said one researcher quoted in the article. "It's now very clear that nurturing the things that you value — whether that's becoming more cultured or redesigning your garden — is what makes people happier."

Buying material goods usually only provides temporary happiness and when you set your sights on acquisition, you often only gain the feeling of wanting more.

"Purchases that support your own values, however, are more satisfying because they help to boost your feelings of self-worth," said the article.

To "get the most bliss for your buck" you have to think long and hard before you spend your money. The article recommends investing in experiences rather than belongings:

"One of the best ways to invest in happiness is to focus on doing rather than owning ... 57 percent (of people asked) said they got more happiness from things they had done — taking a vacation, riding a bike, strolling through a museum, eating a pretzel with a friend — than from stuff they had bought."

It's not only that these activities are fun while we are doing them; it is that we are creating long-lasting memories.

One mother of two interviewed in the article said she has made her financial priorities so they will equal good memories.

"She isn't interested in replacing the television she bought in 1988," the article says. "Instead, she saves her money so she can buy airplane tickets and travel to new places. The jaunts, she says, are exciting stress relievers — even well after they're over and she's back at work: 'I recently spent five days in Paris with my husband, walking down old streets steeped in history. Thinking back on that during an otherwise difficult day relaxes me.'"

These memories will bring her happiness for years to come.

"Material things, on the other hand, quickly lose their luster," this article states. "You may spend hours fantasizing about buying a silk scarf, several days shopping for it and perhaps even some time enjoying it, but not much. Your brain quickly adjusts to the fact that the scarf is folded in your drawer, and before long, you're so used to its being there, you can barely remember when it wasn't.

"Once the object of your obsession, now the scarf blends into the background and becomes as normal to you as hot water, Internet access or automatic-drip coffee."

The article recommends people splurge on mini treats. "It may sound counterintuitive, but researchers have found that over time that small, inexpensive indulgences have virtually the same emotional impact as big, pricey ones — making the little things a much better buy."

Another study examined the purchase of big items versus small ones and the happiness quotient.

"It was the frequent treats of chocolate bars or bottles of wine with takeout dinners that made both groups happy — not the pricier purchase of artwork, designer luggage or CD players."

Click HERE to read more!

Printed in Great Britain
by Amazon